Protecting Your Pets from Parasites

A Holistic Guide to Fleas, Ticks & Heartworms

JUDY MORGAN DVM, CVA, CVCP, CVFT

36 Paws Press

Published by 36 Paws Press
For more information, visit www.drjudymorgan.com

ISBN (paperback): 979-8-9889900-1-7
ISBN (ebook): 979-8-9889900-2-4

Printed in the United States of America

CONTENTS

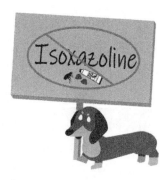

INTRODUCTION

While pests like fleas, ticks and mosquitos can cause diseases in our pets, the new chemicals that are being developed to prevent and treat infestation are extremely toxic, resulting in serious side effects such as seizures, tremors, liver failure, and death. In many cases, a less toxic method of treatment could be undertaken, minimizing risks to our patients.

The use of toxic chemicals to "prevent" fleas, ticks and heartworms taxes your pet's liver and kidneys, which must detoxify the chemicals. Some chemicals stay in the body for the LIFE of your pet. Many chemicals affect the nervous system, causing permanent nerve damage. Many of the chemicals are neurotoxins for insects and ticks, but they can also be neurotoxic to your pet.

By giving heartworm preventatives all year round in cold climates, you are administering unnecessary chemicals. These can also affect the nervous system, along with the liver, kidneys, and immune system. These drugs can cause severe reactions and death when administered along with flea and tick prevention chemicals.

Pet parents are no different than parents with children - it is up to each individual to advocate for their pet and alert their veterinarian to any adverse events or reactions, to question the use of chemicals, and to ask for safer alternatives when they are available. Pet parents are becoming more aware of the dangers associated with parasiticide chemical usage; hopefully this trend will continue for future generations of animals.

FLEAS

Fleas are small bloodsucking insects about 2.5 mm long. While they do not have wings, they can jump long distances, resulting in fleas jumping on your pets and introducing them into your home. Fleas can transfer from animals to humans. The best way to deal with fleas in your environment is to prevent them from entering it in the first place. However, if you suspect or have confirmed you have a flea infestation there are steps you can take to remove them permanently.

Fleas are parasites that love to live on the fur of animals. They can lay up to 50 eggs a day, and up to 2,000 eggs in a female flea's short lifetime. The eggs remain dormant until the temperature and humidity of their environment are optimal for hatching. Fleas are stimulated by vibration and heat. As an example, fleas can remain dormant for months in a vacant property, but after a family moves in, these resilient tiny bugs will seek out a host and start to feed on their blood. There are more than 2,000 species of fleas, some feeding exclusively on certain species of animals. Flea poop is called "flea dirt". Fleas mostly feed around the ears, neck, back, and belly of their host. Fleas seen on your pet represent only 5% of the flea life cycle which includes four stages: eggs, larvae, pupae, and adults.

How do I know if I have a flea problem?

Fleas are not an issue everywhere! The first indication is that your pet will be scratching more than usual. The skin in the location of your pet's scratching can become irritated. A discolored ring around the bite will also signal fleas. Flea bites do not swell like that of a mosquito bite. Your pet's fur may be carrying small black "dots" which look like dirt. Flea bites have a unique bite pattern and location and appear as small, discolored bumps on the skin. The bites often appear in a straight line or a cluster. Your human family members may be scratching as well. Fleas are more likely to bite humans on feet, calves, and ankles.

What diseases can fleas cause in animals?

Flea bite dermatitis is an allergic reaction to flea saliva which leads to intense scratching and itching, allowing the skin to break open and form scabs that can get infected. The most frequent site is the lower back and base of the tail. If an animal continues to scratch at a bite, it can cause swelling, irritation, and welts. Broken skin leads to skin infection and pain. Veterinarians usually prescribe oral, topical, or injected medication to ease irritation and prevent further itching. Unfortunately, steroids and immune-suppressant drugs such as Apoquel are often prescribed. These chemicals come with their own set of side effects which can be deadly and should only be used in extreme cases while trying to solve the underlying problem causing the itch. If an infection has developed, antifungal medication or antibiotics may be prescribed. Antifungal and antibiotic medications destroy the "microbiome" of the gut and skin; the microbiome consists of the beneficial microbes that produce vitamins and fatty acids and contribute to a healthy immune system. Instead of using antibiotic or antifungal treatments, I usually prefer to use a natural, essential-oil shampoo such as those produced by Project Sudz, Kin + Kind, or 4-Legger. Many groomers have a bathing system called Thera-Clean, which can be used to eliminate infections and irritation without the use of chemicals or drugs. The Thera-Clean® System generates Micro-bubbles with a slight negative charge that attract positively charged molecules of dander, sebum, and other organic matter such as dirt, yeast, or bacteria — and even allergens — that can lodge on the hair follicle or clog a pore. The organic matter adheres to the microbubble, which whisks it away. Unlike pressurized cleaning systems, Thera-Clean's water flow is gentle. No soap, shampoo, chemicals, or abrasives are needed. Pets simply sit in a tub with a soft stream of Microbubble-infused water and the Microbubbles do all the work. A thorough cleansing takes only fifteen minutes.

Tapeworms are passed to a pet when the pet ingests a flea that carries tapeworms. This is especially common in pets that self-groom such as cats. Tapeworms cause an itchy rear end as well as weight loss. With-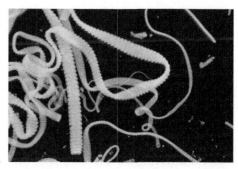out treatment, tapeworms can result in a loss of nutrients and eventually, weight. Severe infestations can result in bowel obstruction. Other symptoms include nausea, weakness, and abdominal pain. If diagnosed with tapeworms, your pet will need treatment. Conventional treatments include anti-parasitic drugs such as praziquantel. Pumpkin seeds are an extremely effective natural deworming agent because they contain a chemical called cucurbitacin. This paralyzes the worms, making them easily eliminated from the intestine. They can be fed whole or ground into a powder. The recommended dose is one teaspoon of raw ground pumpkin seeds per 10lbs of body weight twice a day until the tapeworms are gone. Kanex from Dr. Conor Brady and Parasite Free from Solutions are natural worming supplements.

Flea bite anemia occurs mostly in small animals (puppies and kittens) that have a severe flea infestation. The fleas feed so much on these animals that their red blood cells decrease and they become anemic. Symptoms of flea anemia in dogs and cats include lethargy, poor exercise tolerance, dark stools, dark blood in feces or vomit, pale gums, and skin bruising. To treat anemia, veterinarians may suggest intravenous fluids, antibiotics and in severe cases, blood transfusions. Holistic treatment of anemia includes adding foods to the diet such as egg yolks and sardines, natural blood builders like Amino-B Plex made by Rx Vitamins, and a probiotic with soil-based organisms Humic and Fulvic Acid. The Chinese herb for anemia is called Si Wu Tang or Four Substances.

Cat Scratch Disease (CSD) occurs when fleas pass the bacteria "Bartonella" to cats. Infected cats can then pass the bacteria to other cats or humans through a bite or scratch. Bartonella is associated with numerous conditions including heart disease, eye inflammation, and seizures. The typical signs of CSD are mild fever, chills, and lethargy accompanied by enlarged lymph nodes and lesions on the skin or conjunctiva (the membrane that surrounds the white of the eye and inside of the eyelid). To treat the disease, pets are given antibiotics for six weeks to three months. More serious symptoms include encephalitis (swelling of the brain), fever, and severe muscle pain.

Endemic murine typhus is less common but can occur in warm coastal areas in tropical and subtropical regions. In the US, most cases occur in Southern California and Texas. This disease occurs primarily in rats and mice but can be transmitted to domesticated animals such as cats. Symptoms are like those of distemper and include vomiting, diarrhea (with blood), darkening of the white part of the eye, unusually foul mouth odor, chills, or listlessness. The antibiotic doxycycline is the standard treatment protocol.

Plague is rare in domesticated animals with only a few cases annually reported in the southwestern US. Cats are more susceptible to the plague and are more likely to show clinical signs than dogs. Symptoms include sudden onset fever, chills, headache, nausea, vomiting, abdominal and/or back pain, and weakness. Treatment is achieved through antibiotics.

What flea-borne diseases occur in humans?

Just as in animals, fleas can cause allergies and infections in humans. Small, red itchy bumps will appear when fleas bite humans. Young children are more likely than adults to experience bites and possible infections since they spend more time on the floor. Fleas like to hide in carpets and floor cracks. The key is to reduce the itching and scratching as most infections occur when scratching results in broken skin. Flea bites and itching can be treated with over-the-counter products or home remedies such as antihistamines, hydrocortisone creams, ice, aloe vera, chamomile tea (steep a tea bag for 20 minutes, squeeze it to remove excess water, then apply the bag to the bite). Other remedies include honey, particularly manuka honey (apply topically or take internally), and colloidal oatmeal powder (make a paste with warm water).

Humans can also contract some of the less common flea-borne diseases such as anemia, Cat Scratch Disease (CSD), typhus, and plague. The most common symptoms of these diseases are headache, chills, weakness, nausea, fatigue, and weight loss. If you experience any of these symptoms following flea bites or a home infestation, contact your physician. Most of these diseases are treatable with antibiotics.

How do I eliminate flea infestation?

To deal with a flea infestation, the fleas must be killed at every stage in their life cycle. Since only 5% of the flea life cycle is spent on the pet, the environment must be treated as well as your pets. By focusing only on treating the pet, the problem will remain unresolved.

- A flea comb can be used to remove fleas and flea dirt from your pet. If you find any trace of fleas, remove the collected fleas and fur. Put the fleas in a bowl of dish soap as you remove them, as this will kill them.

- Fleas on pets can be treated with natural shampoos, natural topical treatments, and essential oil sprays. Repeat shampooing weekly until all signs of adult (active) fleas and flea dirt are gone.

- Wash all pet beds, bed coverings, pet clothing, cloth toys, as well as human bedding and clothing with hot water every few days until there are no longer signs of fleas or flea dirt in your home or on your pet. Dry these items on the highest possible heat setting.

- Vacuum carpets thoroughly. Change your vacuum bag immediately. Bagless vacuums should be emptied outside to prevent re-infestation.

- Diatomaceous earth (DE) can be applied to your yard as well as to the pet, pet beds, and carpets. Purchase "food-grade" DE only. DE can irritate the lungs; wear a mask when applying indoors and keep children and pets away until it is thoroughly vacuumed. Repeat the treatment in 4-6 weeks to catch the next batch of younger fleas to prevent another infestation. If using DE on your pet, use small amounts and do not apply to the face, as breathing in the diatoms is harmful to the lungs.

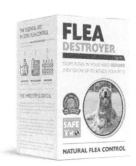

- *Treat your yard and break the cycle where fleas begin using beneficial nematodes.*

- Avoid the use of toxic chemical pesticides, particularly those in the isoxazoline class, as many pets will develop tremors, incoordination, seizures, and may die after application of chemical pesticides.

How do I prevent flea infestation?

Fleas are most active when the weather is warm. They prefer cool, damp areas with a lot of shade. They live around trees, leaves, tall grass, and shrubs. In climates where the temperature dips below freezing, fleas will either be killed or lie dormant until warm weather returns. Those living in warmer climates will find themselves battling fleas all year long. For those living in "4 seasons" climates, September and October are particularly vulnerable as the cooler weather forces fleas indoors. It is suggested flea prevention continue through at least two frosts.

I have made it well-known that I do not recommend or prescribe oral preventative medications that last one to three months, as I feel they are extremely dangerous and have killed too many of our beloved dogs and cats. Even though I have named names in the past, people still send messages and emails daily asking about the use of these products. Once again, I reiterate I do not feel they are safe chemicals that should be fed to our pets or applied topically. Instead, I choose to recommend and use safer, more natural products.

For Cats & Dogs **Dr. Judy's DIY Flea/Tick Spray**

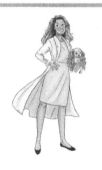

Ingredients:
2 drops lavender essential oil
2 drops lemongrass essential oil
2 drops peppermint essential oil

Directions:
Dilute in 8 ounces of fractionated coconut oil in a spray bottle. Use as needed.

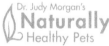

*Avoid eyes, inside ears, and face.

Essential oils have worked well in my hands in the past. Be careful when applying essential oils and don't overdo them. Remember that your pet's sense of smell is much stronger than yours. Apply oils in a well-ventilated area and never spray around the pet's face.

Cedar oil has worked well for many of my clients. It is available for use on pets or in the environment. Not everyone likes the smell of cedar and there are many other essential oil products available. Personally, we use Project Sudz Flea/Tick Spray because I like the smell. Hue and I recently took Project Sudz Flea/Tick Spray with us on our trip to the islands to repel mosquitoes. It worked great! Lavender oil has been shown to repel ticks, while lemongrass oil seems to work particularly well against fleas. Peppermint oil will affect the nervous system of fleas and ticks without harming your pet. Many people use rose geranium oil and find it works well. Neem oil has been around forever and is another favorite. The spray I use for my horses (Ricochet) contains neem and I love the smell. Rose geranium oil is safe to use full strength directly on the pet, but you will only need to apply one drop behind each shoulder blade and one drop near the base of the tail. Other oils should be diluted before applying to pets. Oils can be diluted in fractionated coconut oil and rubbed throughout the coat. They can also be diluted by putting a few drops in your favorite pet shampoo or conditioner. A bandanna with a few drops of diluted essential oil can also be used as a natural flea collar. Make sure the smell is not overwhelming, as this will be close to your dog's nose. Buck Mountain Parasite Dust which contains neem, yarrow, and diatomaceous earth works well too.

Coconut oil kills and repels fleas due to the ingredient lauric acid. Coconut oil can be rubbed through the coat and can be fed to the pets. I use one teaspoon per 20 pounds of body weight twice daily in the food. Coconut oil melts at 76 degrees, so rubbing it between your hands will make it into a liquid that you can rub through your pet's coat. It moisturizes skin and helps kill yeast too.

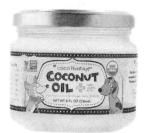

Another great option is garlic. I have used this in the past in my barn for the horses. We still had flies, but the horses eating it were bothered a lot less than the horses that were not. A lot of people claim dogs will die when fed garlic, but that simply is not true. Fresh crushed garlic can also be added to your pet's diet for flea protection. A clove of garlic weighs around five grams. For cats, I recommend up to 1/4 clove (crushed) daily, 3-4 days per week. For dogs, anywhere from 1/2 clove to 2 cloves daily would be considered safe, depending on the size of the dog. A good rule of thumb would be no more than 1/2 clove per 20 pounds of body weight daily, with a maximum of 2 cloves for any size dog. However, if you have a pet that has a history of hemolytic anemia, it would be safer to avoid the use of garlic in any form.

Garlic is not toxic!

Garlic can be beneficial for both dogs and cats in appropriate doses. I use fresh crushed cloves.

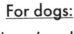

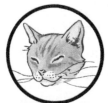

<u>For cats:</u>
1/4 clove (crushed) daily, 3-4 days per week.

<u>For dogs:</u>
1/2 clove (crushed) per 20 pounds of body weight daily, with a maximum of 3 cloves.

Best to take at least 1 day per week off.

I do not recommend using Brewer's Yeast tablets for flea prevention. Brewer's yeast contains B vitamins, but they are processed and degraded. B vitamins supplied naturally through a healthy diet will be more effective.

Beneficial nematodes can be used to kill flea larvae in your yard. Remember, the squirrels, rabbits, mice, and other small critters outside can be harbingers of fleas. Nematodes will not survive in hot, sunny areas of the lawn, but the fleas and ticks do not like those areas either. So spread these little guys in the shady, moist areas where the fleas and ticks are most likely to be found.

Don't forget the old fashioned flea comb. Put the fleas in a bowl of dish soap as you remove them, as this will kill them. These are particularly good for cats because it is a lot harder to bathe a cat. Comb your pets daily if you have any evidence of flea activity.

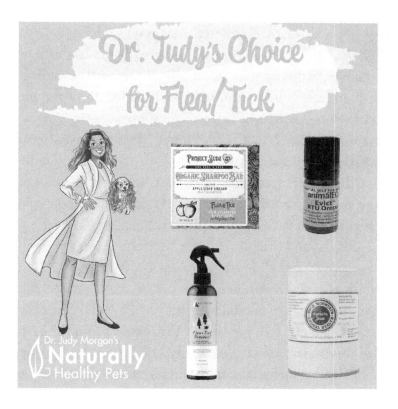

Many people claim vinegar works well. It can be added to the drinking water at the rate of one teaspoon per quart of water. We used to make a mixture of white vinegar and Skin So Soft to use on our horses. They had shiny coats and smelled great! Vinegar can be diluted in water in a 1:1 mixture and sprayed on the coat. I also make my own spray using essential oils and fractionated coconut oil. Make sure you use high quality, pet safe oils. My favorite essential oil supplier for pets is animalEO.

No matter which prevention method you choose, remember that pets can still succumb to diseases spread by these parasites, *even with the use of chemical preventatives.* I have had many patients become ill, even though they had monthly chemicals applied, either topically or orally. Most of the oral and topical products DO NOT REPEL fleas and ticks; they only kill them once they attach to the dog or cat. There are NO guarantees your pet will remain free of pest-borne diseases, no matter what you use.

Vigilance and common sense, along with the use of natural preventatives, will keep your pets healthier overall. By avoiding the use of chemicals, our environment, and the health of the planet for future generations will be greatly improved.

A few years ago, I took a traditional parasite prevention continuing education course. After a discussion of the many flea-borne diseases that are transmissible to our pets and possibly to humans, the conversation turned to the financial impact on veterinary practices that weren't encouraging all pet owners to use year-round heartworm, flea and tick prevention. (Yup, it came down to money.) They analyzed 2.3 million transactions for 263,000 dogs over a 12-month period across ninety-nine practices; the results showed heartworm preventive compliance was just 25% and flea/tick preventive compliance was just 16%. The financial impact on each practice was huge, with an annual opportunity cost per practice of $400,000. Unfortunately, the study did not look at the relevance of:

- practice location

- individual pet exposure to fleas, tick, and heartworms

- environment pets lived in

- travel pets might undergo for significant portions of the year

- individual need for flea, tick, or heartworm prevention

The pharmaceutical companies work diligently to convince the veterinary community that all pets should receive monthly preventative chemicals with no regard to exposure potential. Even veterinary experts, like Dr. Susan Little, a veterinary parasitologist at Oklahoma State University, make blanket statements. Dr. Little and other parasite experts have a mantra: every pet, every month, all year long. According to the OSU website, Dr. Little's laboratory has received research support from the National Institutes of Health, private foundations, and the *veterinary health industry*.I do not feel we should leave the decisions regarding our individual pet's health up to "big pharma". Each pet is an individual and should be treated as such.

TICKS

If you've spent any time outdoors, you and your fur babies have likely encountered ticks at some point. They are attracted to people and their four-legged pets and can move between the two with ease. There are roughly 850 species of ticks around the world. Of these, a handful can carry pathogens which can result in disease for humans or animals.

The following is a primer for identifying the types of ticks that carry disease, how to test a tick for the presence of disease, and how to treat tick bites.

What does a tick bite look like on a dog or cat?

In the absence of finding a tick feeding on its host, a tick bite looks like a small red bump, like a mosquito bite. These bumps often appear at the site of a tick bite or following tick removal and resolve themselves over a few days. Your pet can give you a clue if they are scratching, licking, or chewing the site. If you see persistent scratching, check the hair and the skin in the area. Some tick bites can also produce a "bull's eye" at the bite site.

The best way to check your pet for ticks is to brush your fingers through your pet's fur, applying enough pressure to feel any small bumps. If you feel a bump, pull the fur apart to identify it. An embedded tick will vary in size, from as tiny as a pinhead to as big as a dime. They are usually black, gray or brown. Depending on the size and location of the tick, its legs may also be visible.

To remove a tick, use-fine-tipped tweezers or tick removers to grasp the tick as close to the skin as possible. Clean the area around the bite with witch hazel.

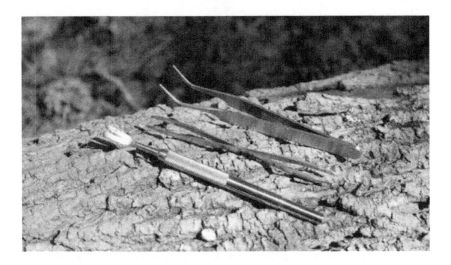

Which tick species are important for dogs and cats?

Tick bites are often harmless and do not cause any symptoms. However, ticks can cause allergic reactions, and certain ticks can pass diseases on to humans and pets when they bite. These diseases can be dangerous or even life threatening when not treated promptly. Ticks are efficient carriers of disease because they attach firmly when sucking blood, feed slowly and may go unnoticed for a considerable time while feeding. Ticks take several days to complete feeding.

Although there are at least fifteen species of ticks in North America, only a few of these species are likely to be encountered by your dog or cat.

TICK BORNE DISEASES

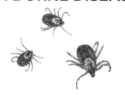

What diseases can ticks transmit to dogs and cats?

Tick-borne diseases are categorized according to the type of bacteria that is transmitted from the tick to its host.

1. *Ehrlichiosis* in dogs is a rickettsial infection caused by the organisms *Ehrlichia canis* and *Ehrlichia lewinii*. The brown dog tick, the Lone Star tick, and the Deer (black-legged) tick spread these bacteria. Rickettsiae are a type of bacteria that inhabit a cell, in this case, the body's white blood cells. This disease is seen throughout the year and throughout the continental United States but is more common on the Gulf Coast, eastern seaboard, Southwest, California, and geographical areas that tend to have an abundance of warm days. Chronic and severe forms of this disease are more representative in Doberman pinschers and German shepherds. Dogs with this infection will show lameness, stiffness, and reluctance to move. The organism lives inside the white blood cells of the dog. It can remain there for months without causing clinical disease symptoms in the dog. Dogs with a healthy immune response will make antibodies against the organism and kill it, resulting in no clinical disease. When symptoms do occur, they may include fever, lethargy, weight loss, swelling of the legs, enlarged lymph

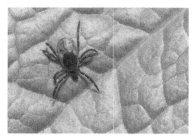

nodes, pale gums, anemia, and seizures. Severe disease can lead to uncontrollable hemorrhage and death.

   a. Testing for Ehrlichiosis includes antibody tests which detect antibodies against the organism in the blood. Antibodies will typically appear seven days after infection. In-office screening tests can have false positive results. Any dog testing positive should have a follow-up PCR test to determine whether *Ehrlichia* organisms are actually present. If the PCR is negative, no treatment is needed, unless the dog is clearly symptomatic.

   b. Treatment includes the use of doxycycline, an antibiotic, once or twice daily for three to four weeks. Improvement should be seen within 24 to 48 hours. Doxycycline commonly causes nausea and vomiting. Doxycycline should not be given with dairy products, as calcium will bind the drug, rendering it useless.

   c. Natural treatment of this disease includes use of the herbs salvia miltiorrhiza (also known as red sage or danshen) and ashwagandha, as well as quercetin, milk thistle, and cordyceps.

   d. No vaccines are available for this disease. Keeping ticks off your dog is your best defense. Please do this as naturally as possible. Your dog's healthy immune system can keep this disease from ever becoming clinically manifested.

2. *Anaplasmosis* is a disease of dogs (and rarely of cats) caused by an infectious organism called *Anaplasma phagocytophilum*. In the United States, Anaplasmosis is most common in

the northeast, upper Midwest, and the west coast. It is an unusual type of bacteria known as rickettsia. The disease is transmitted to dogs and cats by the brown dog tick and the deer (black-legged) tick. Pets with anaplasmosis may never show signs of illness or require

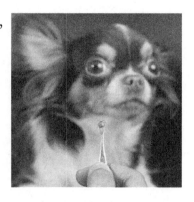

treatment. Those who become ill commonly have a fever, decreased appetite, lethargy, and dehydration. Other signs may include lameness, vomiting and diarrhea, bleeding from the nose, coughing, labored breathing, enlarged lymph nodes, bruising, neck pain, and seizures.

a. Diagnosis is made with a blood test to detect anti-bodies, however false positives may occur. A positive antibody test does not necessarily indicate infection, as antibodies may have formed in response to exposure to the *Anaplasma* bacteria without clinical infection occurring. A PCR, ELISA, or IFA test should be used to confirm infection, as this detects the actual organism in the body. A CBC (complete blood count) should also be performed, as pets with clinical disease will often have thrombocytopenia (low platelet count) and may also be anemic (low red blood cell count).

b. Treatment is the same as that for other closely related tick-borne infections, including Ehrlichiosis and Lyme disease—the antibiotic doxycycline. Most pets are prescribed antibiotics for two to four weeks. Improve-ment should be seen within a few days. If the pet is not markedly improved within 24 to 48 hours, diagnosis and treatment should be re-evaluated. There is no need to retest following treatment, as the antibody test may remain positive for months to years. Treating clinically healthy animals with a positive test is not recommended.

c. Anaplasmosis can infect humans however direct transmission from animals to people or animal to animal is highly unlikely and has not been documented. Dogs, cats, horses, cows, sheep, goats, and humans can be infected.

3. *Rocky Mountain Spotted Fever* is transmitted through tick bites. The species of tick that is involved in transmission varies with the geographical area. In the eastern US, the most common tick to transmit this disease 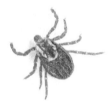 is the American dog tick, and in the western US, the Rocky Mountain wood tick, with the exception of Arizona, where the brown dog tick transmits the disease. In Canada, RMSF is less common but can occur wherever ticks responsible for the transmission of the disease are found. In dogs, the signs of RMSF can be vague and non-specific. Typically, a dog that has become infected may have one or more of the following clinical signs: poor appetite, muscle or joint pain, fever up to 105 degrees, swollen lymph nodes, coughing, abdominal pain, vomiting, diarrhea, swelling of the face or legs, or depression. Focal hemorrhages may occur in the eyes and gums, as well as nosebleeds in severe cases. Neurological signs such as wobbling when walking (ataxia) and painful hypersensitivity can also be seen. In severe cases, where there are a lot of parasites present in the body, extensive damage to blood vessels can cause necrosis (tissue death) of the extremities.

a. Abnormal findings on a complete blood count (CBC) usually include low numbers of platelets (thrombocytopenia) or red blood cells (anemia). In addition, biochemical tests will often show low protein levels, abnormal calcium levels, electrolyte abnormalities, and abnormal liver or kidney values. The gold standard confirmatory test is an Indirect Immunofluorescent Assay (IFA) test. This test requires the submission of two samples of blood; one obtained at the time of illness, and a second test obtained several weeks later. The diagnosis of RMSF is confirmed if the antibody titer increases fourfold between the first and second samples, although a high titer on the first sample can increase suspicion for RMSF. Other tests such as a PCR or a spinal fluid tap can be done but are less sensitive to picking up a diagnosis.

b. Treatment is a course of doxycycline for 7 to 21 days. Enrofloxacin (Baytril) and chloramphenicol can also be used. If RMSF is diagnosed in its early stages and treatment is started immediately, the prognosis for successful treatment is excellent. People and dogs can become infected with RMSF if they are bitten by an infected tick. People cannot get this infection directly from dogs.

4. *Babesiosis* is a rare, sometimes severe, disease caused by the bite of a tick infected with *Babesia microti*, a microscopic protozoal parasite that infects red blood cells. *Babesia* species are found worldwide, although in North America, most cases of babesiosis occur in the southern United States. Babesiosis is considered a serious threat to racing greyhounds and pit bull terriers. Dogs typically present with the acute, severe

form of babesiosis. Cats can be infected through tick bites or bite wounds from infected cats. Symptoms include abnormally dark urine, fever, 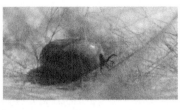 weakness, pale mucous membranes, depression, swollen lymph nodes, and an enlarged spleen.

    a. Blood and urine tests may reveal anemia, thrombocytopenia (low platelets), hypoalbuminemia (low albumin, a blood protein), and bilirubinuria (a pigment from breaking down red blood cells found in the urine).

    b. Conventional treatment for babesiosis includes the antibiotic clindamycin, sometimes in combination with quinine, azithromycin, and atovaquone. The curcumin in turmeric helps alleviate the symptoms of babesiosis. Artemesinin (a derivative of the sweet wormwood plant) helps fight against the babesia parasite. Omega 3 fatty acids can decrease the inflammation associated with the disease.

5. *Powassan Virus Disease*—According to the CDC, approximately 75 cases of Powassan virus disease were reported in the United States over the past **10 years**. Most cases have occurred in the Northeast and Great Lakes region. Signs and symptoms of infection can include fever, headache, vomiting, weakness, confusion, seizures, and memory loss. There is no evidence that this virus affects dogs or cats. That is approximately 7 cases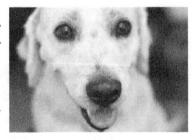

per year in the entire country. However, there have been over **1,000** deaths in dogs from being given isoxazoline-derivative oral flea and tick preventatives in the past **three years.** Rafal Tokarz and his colleagues studied ticks in New York state and found only 1 to 2 percent carried the virus. That is compared to 20 percent carrying the Lyme bacterium, said Tokarz, an associate research scientist at the Center for Infection and Immunity at the Mailman School of Public Health at Columbia University. "If it's 20 percent then your chances are one in five that the tick on you will give you Lyme," he added.

6. *Lyme Disease* is a fast-growing problem around the world. It is caused by the *Borrelia burgdorferi* bacteria. Bites from black-legged ticks or deer ticks can transmit Lyme disease. Symptoms include fever, lethargy, anorexia, lameness, and swollen joints. Secondary heart disease, kidney disease, and seizures may occur. For holistic treatment of Lyme, I use Andrographis, Cat's Claw, Japanese Knotweed, and a medicinal mushroom complex.

LYME DISEASE

Lyme disease, also known as *Lyme borreliosis*, is a bacterial illness that is transmitted by an infected tick to another animal. The spiral-shaped bacterium *Borrelia burgdorferi* carried inside the tick can enter an animal's bloodstream through its bite. Once in the bloodstream, the bacteria can travel to different parts of the body causing problems in specific organs or organ systems, as well as an overall illness. The ticks that carry this type of bacteria are called "black legged" or deer ticks; they are most likely to be found in tall grasses, thick brush, marshes, and woods. Lyme disease occurs in every state in the US, but infection risks vary. Over 95% of cases are from the Northeast, Upper Midwest, and the Pacific Coast. The risk of transmission is highest during 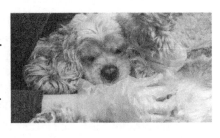 periods when the nymphs (spring) and adults (spring and fall) are actively seeking hosts. Once a tick attaches it may take 1-2 days for it to transmit the bacteria that cause Lyme disease, although recently this has been disputed with many studies pointing to earlier transmission.

What are the symptoms of Lyme disease?

Ninety five percent of dogs infected with the Lyme bacteria remain asymptomatic and do not develop Lyme disease. Even though only a fraction of dogs that carry the bacteria responsible for Lyme disease become ill, pet owners should watch for signs. Symptoms in dogs take 7 to 21 days or even longer following infection to appear. Common symptoms include:

- Painful, swollen joints, causing lameness. Affected dogs have been described as if they were walking on eggshells.

- Fever

- Anorexia (lack of appetite)

- Swollen lymph nodes

- Lethargy

- Depression

Left untreated, canine Lyme disease can damage the heart, nervous system, and kidneys (Lyme nephropathy or Lyme nephritis.)

How are dogs tested and diagnosed for Lyme disease?

There is no single test that can distinguish clinical canine Lyme disease from a simple *Borrelia burgdorferi* infection. When diagnosing Lyme disease, veterinarians make several considerations, including exposure to ticks, signs and symptoms consistent with Lyme disease, as well as other potential diseases. For dogs, blood tests for diagnosing Lyme disease include the Snap 4Dx, Accuplex, C6 test, and the Quant C6 (QC6) test. The C6, Accuplex, and 4Dx tests detect the presence of antibodies created by exposure to the Lyme bacteria. The tests can produce a false negative result if the dog is infected but has not yet formed antibodies or does not form enough antibodies to cause a positive reaction. As such, it is recommended to test no earlier than 4 weeks after a tick bite. The Quant C6 (or QC6) test (such as Cornell University's "Lyme Multiplex" assay) is a follow-up to the other tests; it can be performed to assess the numerical antibody level as confirmation of Lyme disease. Veterinarians may also want to perform a urinalysis before recommending treatment. Dogs shedding protein in their urine are more likely to be actively infected, requiring treatment. One study showed that 40% of dogs diagnosed with Lyme disease were misdiagnosed and had another condition instead.

How is Lyme disease treated?

Because the Lyme spirochete is a bacterium, it can be treated with antibiotics. Lyme disease is usually treated with oral doxycycline for 4 weeks. Other antibiotics such as amoxicillin and azithromycin may be used. The treatment may be extended if symptoms persist. There are several natural alternatives to treat Lyme disease.

- Japanese Knotweed Root—reduces inflammation and Lyme symptoms. It can be used in combination with an antibiotic and is considered a "synergist" meaning that both the herb and the drug will each increase its effectiveness.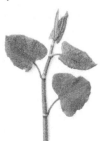

- Cat's Claw—supports the immune system.

- Glucosamine Sulfate—This supplement is often used to help with joint pain and inflammation as well as restoring and protecting cartilage.

- Ledum—a homeopathic remedy used to prevent infection, as well as for the treatment of stiff and painful joints.

- Astragalus—a particularly good immune herb that helps to keep the level of infection low or nonexistent.

- Andrographis—a natural treatment for bacterial infections

The Lyme Vaccine

Lyme vaccinations work to prevent transmission of the *Borrelia* bacteria from the tick to the dog during a tick bite. These vaccines have limitations. They are only 60% to 80% effective in preventing Lyme disease if given prior to the dog being exposed to the disease. They may be less effective in dogs that have already been infected. Some studies indicate that Lyme disease vaccine in dogs may only last about six months, and more studies are needed to confirm these findings. The Lyme vaccine is generally recommended for dogs that live or frequently visit areas known for Lyme disease and high risk of tick exposure. It is never recommended to give a vaccine to a sick dog, even if the dog is sick from Lyme disease. In a study of 1.2 million vaccinated dogs, the Lyme disease vaccine, when used alone, produced more adverse reactions within 3 days than any other canine vaccine. Some studies have shown that vaccination may predispose dogs to inflammation of the kidneys (nephritis) and protein losing nephropathy (PLN) from immune-complex deposition in the kidneys. The vaccine should not be given to dogs living in low-risk areas; some veterinarians question the use of the vaccine for any dog.

Preventing Tick-Borne Diseases

The key to prevention is minimizing your pet's exposure to ticks. There are several preventative measures you can take to help prevent tick-borne disease in your pet.

- Inspect your pets and yourself daily for ticks after walks through the woods or grassy settings. Look especially between toes, on lips, around eyes, inside ears, and under the tail.

- Remove ticks as soon as possible. There are several ways to safely remove a tick from your pet. If desired, take a photo of the tick to show your veterinarian. Ticks can be submitted for testing at TickCheck.com to determine whether they are carrying disease. Be sure to destroy the tick by crushing it before disposing of it.

- Tick prevention products—there are a variety of products used to lower a pet's risk of exposure to ticks. Some can be very toxic to pets and people. I recommend a variety of natural products that are just as effective as the popular conventional tick preventatives.

Ticks like cool, shady places, with dense tall grasses, trees, or shrubs so a short-cut lawn with lots of sun will deter tick infestation. Plant deer resistant plants in your yard so deer will not be as tempted to enter (I found out the hard way they LOVE tulips!). Plant lavender, sage, mint, wormwood, rosemary, and marigolds, which the fleas and ticks do not like. You can also treat your yard with a natural spray or beneficial nematodes.

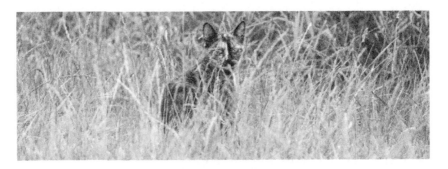

Beneficial nematodes can be used to kill tick larvae in your yard. Food grade Diatomaceous Earth can be sprinkled in the environment or on the pet. Be careful when using DE topically, as you don't want your pet to inhale the dust. DE will be drying to the coat, which is why it works to kill fleas and ticks—it dries them out.

If you are in a suitable area, a few chickens (you can collect your own organic eggs!) or guinea hens will go a long way toward keeping tick populations down to a minimum.

Tickless is an ultrasonic flea & tick repellent safe for pets of all sizes. By fastening the easy-to-use, tiny device onto your cat's or dog's collar, parasites can be kept away for 6-12 months after activation, leaving you and your pet free to enjoy nature. The latest field study suggests the device is 94% efficient against ticks without using any dangerous chemicals!

We use essential oil sprays, as needed, when we will be in high tick areas. Fresh crushed garlic can also be added to your pet's diet for tick protection. For cats, I recommend up to one-fourth clove (crushed) daily, 3-4 days per week. For dogs, anywhere from one-half clove to 2 cloves daily would be considered safe, depending on the size of the dog. An average clove of garlic weighs five grams. A good rule of thumb would be no more than one-half clove per 20 pounds of body weight daily, with a maximum of 2 cloves for any size dog.

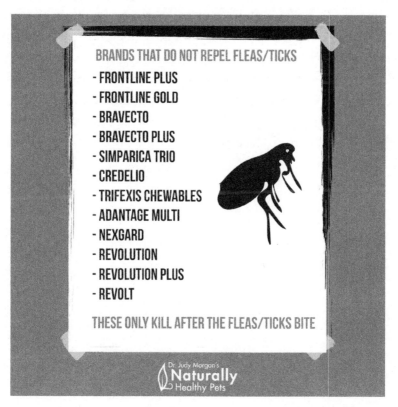

BRANDS THAT DO NOT REPEL FLEAS/TICKS
- FRONTLINE PLUS
- FRONTLINE GOLD
- BRAVECTO
- BRAVECTO PLUS
- SIMPARICA TRIO
- CREDELIO
- TRIFEXIS CHEWABLES
- ADANTAGE MULTI
- NEXGARD
- REVOLUTION
- REVOLUTION PLUS
- REVOLT

THESE ONLY KILL AFTER THE FLEAS/TICKS BITE

Dr. Judy Morgan's
Naturally
Healthy Pets

Most traditional oral and topical chemicals DO NOT REPEL fleas and ticks; they only kill them once they attach to the pet. There are NO guarantees your pet will remain free of pest-borne diseases, no matter what you use.

In heavily infested areas, you may need to stack multiple treatments and prevention methods. When my dogs are at risk of exposure, I use the Tickless tag, Project Sudz Flea/Tick Repel Spray, and a collar with essential oils. I make sure to diligently check myself and my dogs for ticks afterwards using a fine-tooth comb.

This leads to my final point; just because you find one tick on your pet, that does not automatically mean your pet has been exposed to a horrible, deadly disease like Lyme, Ehrlichiosis, Anaplasmosis, Rocky Mountain Spotted Fever, or any number of other tick-borne diseases. As a society, we have been trained to go into panic mode when we see ticks, fleas, mosquitoes, and other pests. We are trained to reach for deadly chemicals JUST IN CASE we might be exposed. Be vigilant, avoid toxic preventatives, and choose safer, natural options. Ticks can be submitted for testing at TickCheck.com to show if they are carrying disease if you want to know more.

HEARTWORMS

Heartworm disease in dogs is a global problem. The domestic dog and wild canids are the main hosts, however infection in cats and other species has occasionally been reported.

Transmission

Mosquitoes are the main vector of transmission. The first three stages of larvae develop in mosquitoes. Historically, it was taught that L1 and L2 larvae require temperatures above 57 F (14 C) for a minimum of two weeks to reach L3, the infective stage, however this has recently been raised to 80 degrees Fahrenheit Therefore, transmission may be seasonal in some areas, but most veterinarians recommend year-round administration of heartworm preventative medications. (I am not one of those veterinarians.)

The infective L3 larvae molt to L4 over a couple of weeks in the dog and then mature into L5, which are immature adults, over a 45 to 60 day period in the muscles. The L5 larvae then enter the bloodstream to be carried to the heart and pulmonary artery where they mature over four to five months. After approximately seven months, the mature adults produce microfilariae that enter the circulation.

Diagnosis

Dogs usually show no signs of illness until adult worms are present in the heart. Clinical signs include cough, exercise intolerance, labored respiration, weight loss, fainting, coughing up blood, and congestive heart failure. Interestingly, vomiting is a common sign in cats.

Blood tests are used to detect antigen from female heartworms. False negative test results are possible if there are only male worms present, there is a sparse number of female worms, or the worms are immature. Blood smears under the microscope may show swimming microfilariae.

Chest X-rays are the best method for determining the severity of disease. Echocardiograms may show worms present in the heart and main pulmonary artery. Laboratory testing may show changes in liver and kidney function.

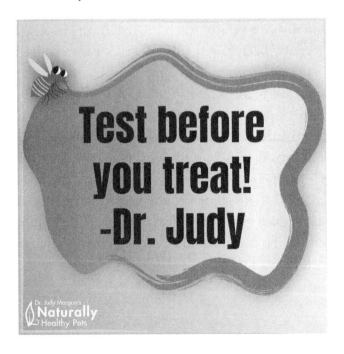

Treatment

The goal of treatment is to eliminate adult worms, microfilariae, and any migrating L3, L4, and L5 larvae. The only FDA approved drug to kill adult worms is Melarsomine Dihydrochloride. Treatment consists of three injections deep into the lumbar (lower back) muscles. One injection is followed by two injections given 24 hours apart one month later. Exercise restriction is essential during this two-month period, as death of the worms can result in pulmonary thromboembolism (blood clots in the lungs).

Steroids are prescribed to help decrease inflammation from worm death and the clinical effects of thromboembolism.

Doxycycline (antibiotic) is prescribed prior to the melarsomine injections. Doxycycline has been shown to kill L3 and L4. It also kills the *Wolbachia* bacteria found in adult heartworms that help them survive. Heartworm preventative medications such as oral ivermectin and milbemycin oxime, topical moxidectin and selamectin, and injectable slow release moxidectin are also started two months prior to melarsomine injections. This is to ensure L3 and L4 larvae will not continue to mature. Moxidectin has significant side effects and is not recommended. Monthly oral ivermectin and milbemycin oxime are much safer and recommended for use over moxidectin.

Side effects from the melarsomine injection can include: (from drug.com)

ADVERSE REACTIONS (SIDE EFFECTS): Injection Sites: At the recommended dosage in clinical field trials, significant irritation was observed at the intramuscular injection sites, accompanied by pain, swelling, tenderness, and reluctance to move. Approximately 30% of treated dogs experienced some kind of reaction at the injection site(s). Though injection site reactions were generally mild to moderate in severity and recovery occurred in 1 week to 1 month, severe reactions did occur (< 1.0 %), so care should be taken to avoid superficial or subcutaneous injection and leakage. Firm nodules can persist indefinitely.

Other Reactions: Coughing/gagging, depression/lethargy, anorexia/inappetence, fever, lung congestion, and vomiting were the most common reactions observed in dogs. Hypersalivation and panting occurred rarely in clinical trials (1.9% and 1.6%, respectively); however, these signs may occur within 30 minutes of injection and may be severe. One dog vomited after each injection. All adverse reactions resolved with time or treatment with the exception of a limited number of injection site reactions (persistent nodules) and a low number of post-treatment deaths.

An alternative to this "quick kill" method is the "slow kill" method. The slow kill method involves use of Doxycycline for one month, then two months off, then repeat for a period of one year (4 cycles). Monthly preventatives are also administered during the year. Most dogs will clear the infection within one year. I have had success with this method with many patients. Traditional veterinarians generally do not like to employ this method. Dogs must lead a sedentary lifestyle until the worms are cleared.

Preventing Heartworms

Preventatives such as oral ivermectin and milbemycin oxime, topical moxidectin and selamectin, and injectable slow release moxidectin (Proheart 6 and Proheart 12) do not prevent mosquitoes from biting the pet; they kill the L3 and L4 larvae, as well as microfilariae if they are present. I do not recommend using moxidectin or selamectin due to the high number of adverse reactions and death that have occurred. If I had to choose the least of the evils, milbemycin oxime would be my preferred drug.

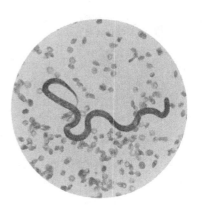

Healthy dogs with a good immune system are less likely to develop overwhelming heartworm infections. It is important to feed a whole-food, human-grade diet. Proper exercise, lean body weight, and immune-support will go a long way to keeping your dog parasite-free.

As a holistic veterinarian I am often asked which natural preventative I recommend for heartworm prevention. This is always a tricky question because there are so many variables that come into play. While there are websites that warn against the use of any and all chemicals in or on our pets, I often question whether it is possible in all environments to have our pets remain completely chemical-free. It is a great goal, but we must face the realities of the polluted world in which we live, creating daily health stressors that contribute to compromised immune function.

Factors to consider when deciding whether to give heartworm prevention might include:

- Environmental temperature: Heartworms are spread by mosquitoes. A female mosquito must bite an infected canine. The immature larvae are ingested and live in the salivary glands of the mosquito where they mature in about two weeks (at 80F), as long as the environmental temperature remains above 57 degrees Fahrenheit around the clock. There are some areas of the world where the temperatures do not remain warm enough for a long enough period of time to allow this process to occur.

- There must be a reservoir of infected canines for mosquitoes to feed on.

- Mosquitoes survive best in high humidity.

- Most cases of heartworm occur in the Mississippi River Valley and southeastern United States.

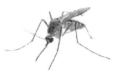

There are many natural ways to minimize mosquito populations:

- Use natural mosquito repellents.

- Bats and purple martins eat very few mosquitoes. The main predators of mosquitoes are fish and dragonflies.

- Eliminate standing water. Mosquitoes spend the first ten days of their life in water.

- Bacteria can be used to kill mosquito larvae. *Bacillus thuringiensis israelensis* (Bti) is a commercially produced bacteria, sold in pellet and powder form, that can be laced into water where larvae live. It produces proteins that turn into toxins after the larvae eat it.

- Dark clothing attracts mosquitoes, as will dark coats on animals. Light-weight white fly netting can be used to keep mosquitoes away (commonly used as horse blankets to keep flies away in summer).

- Mosquito traps with attractants can kill thousands of mosquitoes per night.

A healthy dog with a healthy immune system will have decreased risk of development of adult heartworms, a process that takes seven to nine months from the time the mosquito bites. A healthy immune system will recognize heartworm larvae as foreign invaders, mounting an attack that can successfully defeat the invasion. Unfortunately, very few dogs have a fully functioning healthy immune system due to over-vaccination, over-use of medications and chemicals, and poor quality nutrition found in many commercial diets.

Do not blindly accept the recommendation to give preventative chemicals year-round if you live in an area that has cold winters. I do not recommend giving heartworm prevention chemicals if the temperatures drop significantly in certain seasons. Heartworm larvae need to mature for two weeks in the salivary glands of the mosquito. If the ambient temperature drops below 57 degrees at any time during that period, the larvae stop maturing. So, until the temperature remains above 57 degrees for two weeks straight (including overnight), I do not worry about heartworms being spread. I do not give my dogs heartworm prevention. My daughter's dogs that spend more time outside will get a preventative every 45 days until two to four weeks after the temperature starts

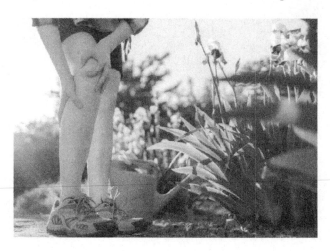

to stay consistently below 57 in the fall (usually November).

Do not be swayed by pharmaceutical companies trying to sell more drugs. Treat your pets as needed, based on where you live. The number of positive cases in the extremely hot southern parts of our country are high. Unfortunately, there are also areas in the south where veterinary care is not a high priority, which means the reservoir of positive dogs that mosquitoes can bite is much higher.

If you are considering skipping heartworm prevention, make sure you know the facts about heartworm prevalence in your area. In my clinic the only preventative we carried was Interceptor, which contains milbemycin. Some clients opt for Sentinel, which also contains lufeneron, which prevents flea eggs from hatching. I do NOT recommend using Interceptor PLUS or Sentinel SPEC-TRUM, which also contain a tapeworm dewormer, praziquantel. Unless your pet has chronic flea infestation, they will not have

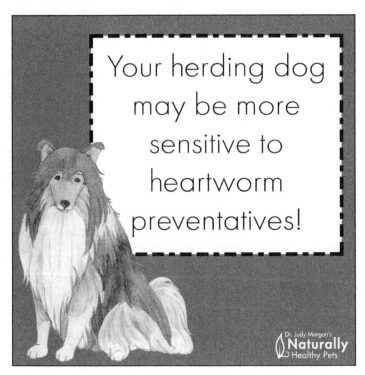

chronic tapeworm infestation. Beware of products containing Moxidectin (Proheart 6 and Proheart 12), a particularly dangerous chemical dewormer. Long-acting injections may seem convenient, but once given, there is no antidote to reverse side effects which may include the following adverse reactions: anaphylaxis, vomiting, diarrhea (with and without blood), listlessness, weight loss, seizures, and death. Any dogs with the MDR1 gene mutation typically found in herding breeds should avoid Ivermectin. It is one of the drugs they are commonly sensitive to.

If you want to be like me and avoid using toxic chemicals on your dog in the name of heartworm prevention all together, I recommend Vital Animals Don't Get Heartworm by Will Falconer, DVM

AVOIDING SPOOKY DRUGS

I avoid the following parasiticides due to their high rate of adverse reactions and long term, negative effects: Isoxazolines (Bravecto, Credelio, Nexgard, Simparica, Revolution Plus), Moxidectin (Proheart 6 or 12, Advantage Multi), Fipronil (Frontline, PetArmor Plus), Spinosad with Milbemycin (Trifexis), Selamectin (Revolution), and Imidacloprid and Flumethrin (Seresto).

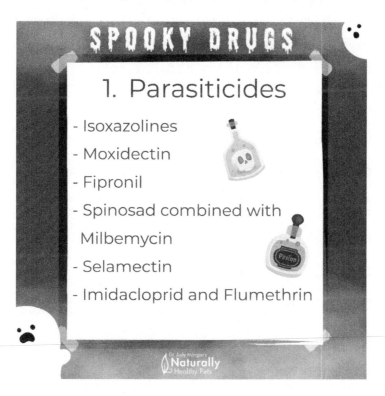

Isoxazoline based products used for prevention and treatment of fleas, ticks, and mites (Bravecto, Bravecto Plus, Nexgard, Simparica, Simparica Trio, Credelio, Revolution Plus) are gaining popularity. Many traditional (and even some holistic) veterinarians are strongly recommending the use of the isoxazoline class of products. Unfortunately, as the number of animals being given these products has risen, so has the number of pet owners reporting neurological and other adverse reactions.

What side effects are possible when using these drugs?

Neurological side effects or adverse reactions can range from barely noticeable to severe. Adverse reactions to these compounds appear to affect animals randomly, although those with certain chronic diseases, the young and elderly, animals that are immune-compromised, or those that have the genetic mutation of the MDR1 gene seem to be at higher risk. A survey of pet owners showed that adverse reactions are common.

Some adverse reactions that my clients have seen include:

- Aggression
- Personality changes
- Seizures
- Disorientation
- Wobbling or unstable gate
- Sensitivity to touch
- Abnormal vocalizations
- Urinary or fecal incontinence
- Death

I have seen these adverse reactions happen immediately after administration, but I have also worked with cases where the pet parent noticed these reactions days, weeks, or even months later. Sometimes the reactions do not occur until multiple doses of the medication have been given, as the medications build up in the body.

Other side effects that have been reported include:

- Liver failure

- Kidney failure

- Dry eye

- Clotting disorders

- Internal hemorrhage

- Skin disease and itching

- Vomiting

- Diarrhea

- Inappetence

- Drooling

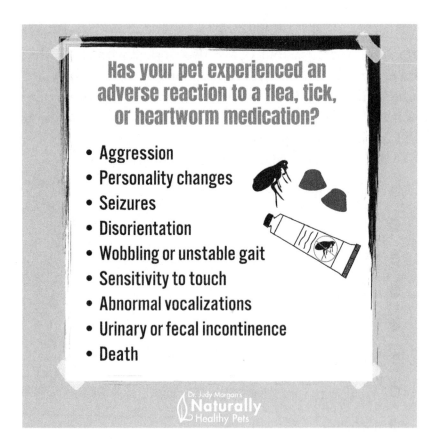

What should I do if I believe my pet is having an adverse reaction?

First and foremost, take your pet to the veterinarian immediately if you believe your animal is having an adverse reaction. Many pet owners like that some of these products come in tablet form which makes for easy administration. The problem with this form of administration (oral ingestion) with any medication is that once something is ingested by the animal, it cannot be removed easily unless the patient is presented within an hour of dosing. In my clinics, I did see some emergency cases where a pet would come in experiencing a severe reaction to a **topical** flea or tick medication; in those cases, one piece of my treatment protocol would be bathing the animal to remove as much of the medication as possible. We do not have this option with medications that are given orally.

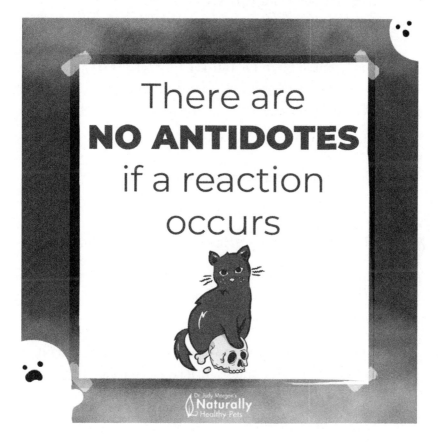

These animals need to have their liver and kidneys detoxed, then supported. In my book, Yin & Yang Nutrition for Dogs, you can use the Liver Support, Liver Draining, Blood Tonic, and Kidney diets.

I also suggest the following supplements:

- Milk Thistle 50-100mg per 25lbs twice daily (you can also use Hepato Support made by Rx Vitamins or Liver Tonic made by Adored Beast)

- NAC (N-acetylcysteine) 500mg twice daily for 2 weeks then once daily for two weeks

- Chlorella 25mg twice daily for 3 weeks

- The Chinese Herb Di Tan Tang for seizures 0.5 gm per 20 pounds body weight twice daily until the pet has been free of seizures for at least three months

- Liposomal Glutathione 100mg daily for a week

- Curcumin 100mg once daily for a week

- Broccoli Sprouts 100mg once daily for a week

- Gaba Aminobutyric Acid 100mg once daily for a week

- Add asparagus and dandelion greens or root to the diet. Dark leafy greens such as kale, beet tops, and spinach may be helpful.

- Epsom salt/baking soda baths to pull out toxins daily for fifteen to twenty minutes in very warm water

- MCT oil one teaspoon per twenty pounds body weight twice daily with food

Some pet parents have continued these supplements for longer periods of time with no adverse effects if the pet is still experiencing symptoms.

Report the incident to the FDA and the manufacturer!

It is also important to report the adverse reactions to the FDA and the manufacturer of the medication that was given. The FDA continues to monitor adverse drug event reports for these products and encourages pet owners and veterinarians to report adverse drug events. You can do this by reporting to the drugs' manufacturers, who are required to report this information to the FDA, or by submitting a report directly to the FDA.

- 🐾 To report suspected adverse drug events for these products and/or obtain a copy of the Safety Data Sheet (SDS) or for technical assistance, contact the appropriate manufacturers at the following phone numbers:
    - Merck Animal Health (Bravecto, Bravecto Plus): 800-224-5318
    - Elanco Animal Health (Credelio, Seresto, Trifexis): 888-545-5973
    - Boehringer Ingelheim (Nexgard, Frontline): 888-637-4251
    - Zoetis (Simparica, Simparica Trio, Revolution Plus, Proheart): 888-963-8471

- 🐾 If you prefer to report directly to the FDA, or want additional information about adverse drug experience reporting for animal drugs, see How to Report Animal Drug and Device Side Effects and Product Problems.

- 🐾 Pet owners and veterinarians who have additional questions can contact AskCVM@fda.hhs.gov or call 240-402-7002.

What are the long term effects?

With the cases I have seen so far, some animals are able to make a full recovery while others will experience side effects indefinitely. Using my protocol, I have been able to help improve the quality of life of many animals, but it is important to remember that the damage done may be permanent. Some of my clients now must deal with seizures or other neurological side effects for the rest of their pet's life.

With any animal that had any level of neurological or internal adverse reaction to these medications, I recommend keeping them as far away from chemicals as possible for the rest of their lives. This means using natural flea and tick prevention, asking for vaccine titers (blood tests to determine whether your pet has immunity to disease), or getting exemptions instead of vaccinations. These pets need to be fed a high-quality, species-appropriate diet made with human-grade ingredients.